VEGAN DIABETIC RENAL DIET COOKBOOK

COOKBOOK

A Comprehensive Cookbook for Plant-based Delights

Dr Lily Morgan

COPYRIGHT PAGE

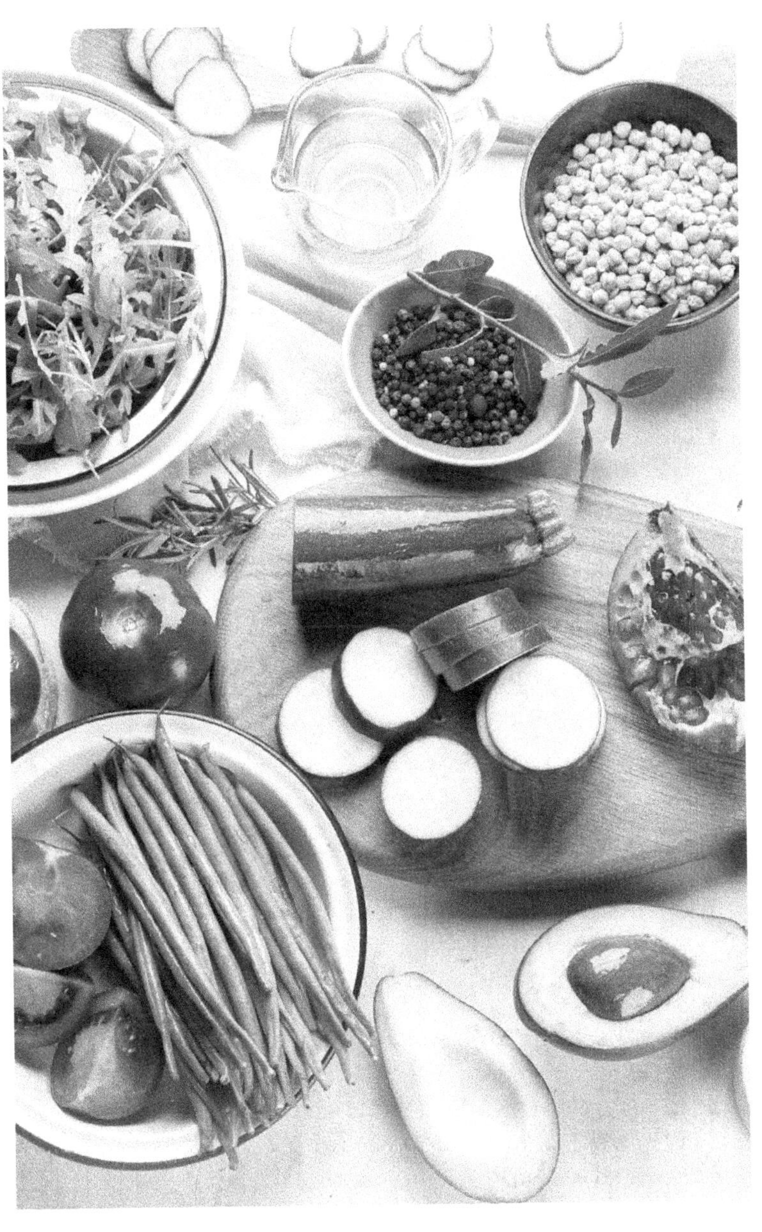

TABLE OF CONTENTS

INTRODUCTION

I n today's world, where health concerns and dietary restrictions are becoming increasingly prevalent, it is essential to have access to specialized cookbooks that cater to specific needs. The "Vegan Diabetic Renal Diet Cookbook" is a valuable resource designed to assist individuals following a vegan diet while managing diabetes and renal health. This chapter serves as an introduction to the cookbook, providing an overview of its purpose, the importance of understanding diabetes and renal health, the benefits of a vegan diet, and guidelines for following the diet effectively.

About the Vegan Diabetic Renal Diet Cookbook

The "Vegan Diabetic Renal Diet Cookbook" is a comprehensive guide filled with delicious and nutritious recipes tailored specifically for individuals who adhere to a vegan lifestyle while dealing with diabetes and renal concerns. This cookbook aims to provide creative and flavorful meal options that prioritize both health and taste. With a wide array of breakfasts, lunches, dinners, snacks, appetizers, and desserts, this cookbook offers a diverse range of recipes to suit different preferences and dietary requirements.

Understanding Diabetes and Renal Health

Before diving into the intricacies of the vegan diabetic renal diet, it is crucial to comprehend the underlying conditions of diabetes and renal health. Diabetes is a chronic metabolic disorder characterized by high blood sugar levels, resulting from insufficient insulin production or ineffective insulin utilization. Renal health, on the other hand, refers to the well-being of the kidneys, which play a vital role in filtering waste products from the blood.

Benefits of a Vegan Diabetic Renal Diet

Adopting a vegan diet can provide numerous benefits for individuals managing diabetes and renal health. A vegan diet emphasizes plant-based foods, such as fruits, vegetables, whole grains, legumes, nuts, and seeds, while avoiding animal products and by-products. This dietary approach can help regulate blood sugar levels, reduce the risk of cardiovascular disease, improve kidney function, promote weight management, and enhance overall health and well-being.

Guidelines for Following the Diet

To reap the maximum benefits of the vegan diabetic renal diet, it is important to understand and follow specific guidelines. This section of the chapter outlines key principles for successfully implementing the diet:

Monitoring Carbohydrate Intake: Carbohydrates have a direct impact on blood sugar levels. Understanding portion sizes and choosing complex carbohydrates with a low glycemic index can help maintain stable blood sugar levels.

Controlling Protein Intake: As renal health may be compromised in individuals with diabetes, monitoring protein intake is crucial. The cookbook provides recipes with appropriate protein sources that are beneficial for renal health.

Managing Sodium Intake: Sodium can contribute to hypertension and fluid retention. The cookbook focuses on using herbs, spices, and other flavor-enhancing ingredients to reduce the need for excessive salt.

Balancing Healthy Fats: While fats should be consumed in moderation, incorporating healthy fats, such as avocados, nuts, and seeds, can provide essential nutrients and promote satiety.

Adequate Fluid Intake: Staying well-hydrated is important for kidney health. The cookbook suggests refreshing and hydrating beverage options to help individuals meet their fluid needs.

Regular Physical Activity: Alongside dietary modifications, engaging in regular physical activity is encouraged. The cookbook highlights the importance of incorporating exercise into a healthy lifestyle.

Kitchen Essentials and Ingredient Substitutions

Equipping your kitchen with the necessary tools and ingredients is essential for successfully preparing the recipes in the cookbook. This section provides an overview of kitchen essentials, such as quality knives, cutting boards, measuring utensils, and cooking appliances. Additionally, it suggests ingredient substitutions for individuals with specific dietary restrictions or preferences, ensuring that the recipes can be adapted to suit various needs.

Tips for Meal Planning and Preparation

Efficient meal planning and preparation are fundamental for maintaining a healthy and consistent dietary routine. This section offers practical tips and strategies for meal planning, including creating shopping lists, batch cooking, and utilizing leftovers. It also provides advice on efficient meal preparation, such as prepping ingredients in advance, utilizing time-saving cooking techniques, and storing meals properly to maintain freshness and taste.

Chapter 1: 30 Day Meal Plan

Week 1

Day 1:

Breakfast: Quinoa Porridge with Berries and Almonds

Lunch: Lentil and Vegetable Soup

Dinner: Baked Tofu with Roasted Vegetables

Snack: Roasted Chickpeas with Spices

Dessert: Vegan Chocolate Avocado Mousse

Day 2:

Breakfast: Tofu Scramble with Vegetables

Lunch: Mexican Quinoa Salad with Lime Dressing

Dinner: Spaghetti Squash with Tomato Basil Sauce

Snack: Guacamole with Baked Tortilla Chips

Dessert: Berry and Coconut Chia Seed Pudding

Day 3:

Breakfast: Avocado Toast with Lemon and Sprouts

Lunch: Chickpea and Vegetable Stir-Fry

Dinner: Vegan Pad Thai with Tofu and Vegetables

Snack: Vegan Spinach Artichoke Dip

Dessert: Baked Apples with Cinnamon and Walnuts

Day 4:

Breakfast: Buckwheat Pancakes with Sugar-Free Berry
Compote

Lunch: Kale and White Bean Salad with Lemon Vinaigrette

Dinner: Stuffed Portobello Mushrooms with Quinoa and
Spinach

Snack: Carrot and Hummus Sticks

Dessert: Vegan Pumpkin Pie Bars

Day 5:

Breakfast: Chia Pudding with Coconut Milk and Mango

Lunch: Roasted Vegetable Wrap with Hummus

Dinner: Moroccan Chickpea Stew with Couscous

Snack: Oven-Baked Sweet Potato Fries

Dessert: Coconut Rice Pudding with Mango

Day 6:

Breakfast: Lentil and Vegetable Breakfast Bowl

Lunch: Sweet Potato and Black Bean Chili

Dinner: Ratatouille with Quinoa Pilaf

Snack: Cucumber Sushi Rolls with Avocado

Dessert: Vegan Banana Ice Cream with Peanut Butter

Day 7:

Breakfast: Green Smoothie with Spinach, Kale, and Apple

Lunch: Mediterranean Stuffed Bell Peppers

Dinner: Vegan Lentil Loaf with Mashed Cauliflower

Snack: Spicy Edamame

Dessert: Lemon Poppy Seed Energy Balls

Week 2

Day 8:

Breakfast: Chickpea Flour Omelet with Sautéed Vegetables

Lunch: Vegan Sushi Rolls with Quinoa and Avocado

Dinner: Coconut Curry with Chickpeas and Brown Rice

Snack: Mediterranean Stuffed Grape Leaves

Dessert: Chocolate Chip Oatmeal Cookies

Day 9:

Breakfast: Overnight Oats with Almond Milk and
Cinnamon

Lunch: Spinach and Lentil Salad with Balsamic Dressing

Dinner: Zucchini Noodles with Creamy Cashew Sauce

Snack: Vegan Nachos with Cashew Cheese

Dessert: Almond Butter Cups

Day 10:

Breakfast: Sweet Potato Hash Browns with Tofu Bacon

Lunch: Mushroom and Barley Soup

Dinner: Black Bean and Vegetable Enchiladas

Snack: Roasted Red Pepper and Walnut Dip

Dessert: Blueberry Crumble Bars

Day 11:

Breakfast: Vegan Banana Bread with Walnuts

Lunch: Curried Chickpea Salad Wraps

Dinner: Stuffed Bell Peppers with Quinoa and Black Beans

Snack: Crispy Baked Tofu Bites

Dessert: Vegan Carrot Cake with Cream Cheese Frosting

Day 12:

Breakfast: Spinach and Mushroom Breakfast Burrito

Lunch: Quinoa and Black Bean Burgers

Dinner: Teriyaki Tofu Stir-Fry with Brown Rice

Snack: Stuffed Mushrooms with Herbed Quinoa

Dessert: Raspberry Coconut Bliss Balls

Day 13:

Breakfast: Quinoa and Vegetable Breakfast Muffins

Lunch: Cauliflower Fried Rice

Dinner: Creamy Vegan Alfredo Pasta with Broccoli

Snack: Baked Kale Chips with Sea Salt

Dessert: Matcha Green Tea Popsicles

Day 14:

Breakfast: Quinoa Porridge with Berries and Almonds

Lunch: Lentil and Vegetable Soup

Dinner: Baked Tofu with Roasted Vegetables

Snack: Roasted Chickpeas with Spices

Dessert: Vegan Chocolate Avocado Mousse

Week 3

Day 15:

Breakfast: Tofu Scramble with Vegetables

Lunch: Mexican Quinoa Salad with Lime Dressing

Dinner: Spaghetti Squash with Tomato Basil Sauce

Snack: Guacamole with Baked Tortilla Chips

Dessert: Berry and Coconut Chia Seed Pudding

Day 16:

Breakfast: Avocado Toast with Lemon and Sprouts

Lunch: Chickpea and Vegetable Stir-Fry

Dinner: Vegan Pad Thai with Tofu and Vegetables

Snack: Vegan Spinach Artichoke Dip

Dessert: Baked Apples with Cinnamon and Walnuts

Day 17:

Breakfast: Buckwheat Pancakes with Sugar-Free Berry

Compote

Lunch: Kale and White Bean Salad with Lemon Vinaigrette

Dinner: Stuffed Portobello Mushrooms with Quinoa and

Spinach

Snack: Carrot and Hummus Sticks

Dessert: Vegan Pumpkin Pie Bars

Day 18:

Breakfast: Chia Pudding with Coconut Milk and Mango

Lunch: Roasted Vegetable Wrap with Hummus

Dinner: Moroccan Chickpea Stew with Couscous

Snack: Oven-Baked Sweet Potato Fries

Dessert: Coconut Rice Pudding with Mango

Day 19:

Breakfast: Lentil and Vegetable Breakfast Bowl

Lunch: Sweet Potato and Black Bean Chili

Dinner: Ratatouille with Quinoa Pilaf

Snack: Cucumber Sushi Rolls with Avocado

Dessert: Vegan Banana Ice Cream with Peanut Butter

Day 20:

Breakfast: Green Smoothie with Spinach, Kale, and Apple

Lunch: Mediterranean Stuffed Bell Peppers

Dinner: Vegan Lentil Loaf with Mashed Cauliflower

Snack: Spicy Edamame

Dessert: Lemon Poppy Seed Energy Balls

Day 21:

Breakfast: Chickpea Flour Omelet with Sautéed Vegetables

Lunch: Vegan Sushi Rolls with Quinoa and Avocado

Dinner: Coconut Curry with Chickpeas and Brown Rice

Snack: Mediterranean Stuffed Grape Leaves

Dessert: Chocolate Chip Oatmeal Cookies

Week 4

Day 22:

Breakfast: Overnight Oats with Almond Milk and Cinnamon

Lunch: Spinach and Lentil Salad with Balsamic Dressing

Dinner: Zucchini Noodles with Creamy Cashew Sauce

Snack: Vegan Nachos with Cashew Cheese

Dessert: Almond Butter Cups

Day 23:

Breakfast: Sweet Potato Hash Browns with Tofu Bacon

Lunch: Mushroom and Barley Soup

Dinner: Black Bean and Vegetable Enchiladas

Snack: Roasted Red Pepper and Walnut Dip

Dessert: Blueberry Crumble Bars

Day 24:

Breakfast: Vegan Banana Bread with Walnuts

Lunch: Curried Chickpea Salad Wraps

Dinner: Stuffed Bell Peppers with Quinoa and Black Beans

Snack: Crispy Baked Tofu Bites

Dessert: Vegan Carrot Cake with Cream Cheese Frosting

Day 25:

Breakfast: Spinach and Mushroom Breakfast Burrito

Lunch: Quinoa and Black Bean Burgers

Dinner: Teriyaki Tofu Stir-Fry with Brown Rice

Snack: Stuffed Mushrooms with Herbed Quinoa

Dessert: Raspberry Coconut Bliss Balls

Day 26:

Breakfast: Quinoa and Vegetable Breakfast Muffins

Lunch: Cauliflower Fried Rice

Dinner: Creamy Vegan Alfredo Pasta with Broccoli

Snack: Baked Kale Chips with Sea Salt

Dessert: Matcha Green Tea Popsicles

Day 27:

Breakfast: Quinoa Porridge with Berries and Almonds

Lunch: Lentil and Vegetable Soup

Dinner: Baked Tofu with Roasted Vegetables

Snack: Roasted Chickpeas with Spices

Dessert: Vegan Chocolate Avocado Mousse

Day 28:

Breakfast: Tofu Scramble with Vegetables

Lunch: Mexican Quinoa Salad with Lime Dressing

Dinner: Spaghetti Squash with Tomato Basil Sauce

Snack: Guacamole with Baked Tortilla Chips

Dessert: Berry and Coconut Chia Seed Pudding

Day 29:

Breakfast: Avocado Toast with Lemon and Sprouts

Lunch: Chickpea and Vegetable Stir-Fry

Dinner: Vegan Pad Thai with Tofu and Vegetables

Snack: Vegan Spinach Artichoke Dip

Dessert: Baked Apples with Cinnamon and Walnuts

Day 30:

Breakfast: Buckwheat Pancakes with Sugar-Free Berry
Compote

Lunch: Kale and White Bean Salad with Lemon Vinaigrette

Dinner: Stuffed Portobello Mushrooms with Quinoa and Spinach

Snack: Carrot and Hummus Sticks

Dessert: Vegan Pumpkin Pie Bars

Congratulations on completing the 30-day meal plan! You've successfully explored a variety of delicious and nutritious vegan diabetic renal recipes

Chapter 2: Breakfast Recipes

In this chapter, we will explore a variety of delicious and nutritious vegan breakfast recipes that are suitable for individuals following a diabetic renal diet. These recipes are carefully crafted to provide a balance of essential nutrients while considering the dietary restrictions and health needs of individuals with diabetes and renal issues.

Quinoa Porridge with Berries and Almonds

Ingredients:

- 1/2 cup quinoa
- 1 cup unsweetened almond milk
- 1 cup mixed berries (such as strawberries, blueberries, and raspberries)
- 2 tablespoons sliced almonds
- 1 tablespoon maple syrup (optional)
- 1/2 teaspoon vanilla extract
- Pinch of cinnamon

Instructions:

1. Rinse the quinoa thoroughly under cold water.
2. In a medium saucepan, combine the rinsed quinoa and almond milk. Bring to a boil over medium heat.
3. Reduce the heat to low, cover the saucepan, and simmer for 15-20 minutes, or until the quinoa is cooked and the mixture has thickened.
4. Remove the saucepan from the heat and stir in the vanilla extract and cinnamon.
5. Divide the quinoa porridge into bowls and top with mixed berries and sliced almonds.
6. Drizzle with maple syrup if desired. Enjoy warm.

Tofu Scramble with Vegetables

Ingredients:

- 1 tablespoon olive oil
- 1/2 block firm tofu, crumbled
- 1/4 cup diced onion
- 1/4 cup diced bell peppers
- 1/4 cup diced tomatoes
- 1/4 cup diced zucchini
- 1/4 teaspoon turmeric

- 1/4 teaspoon garlic powder
- 1/4 teaspoon onion powder
- Salt and pepper to taste
- Fresh parsley, for garnish

Instructions:

1. Heat the olive oil in a skillet over medium heat.
2. Add the crumbled tofu, diced onion, bell peppers, tomatoes, and zucchini to the skillet. Sauté for 5-7 minutes until the vegetables are tender.
3. Sprinkle turmeric, garlic powder, onion powder, salt, and pepper over the tofu and vegetables. Stir well to combine and cook for another 2-3 minutes.
4. Remove from heat and garnish with fresh parsley. Serve hot.

Avocado Toast with Lemon and Sprouts

Ingredients:

- 2 slices whole grain bread
- 1 ripe avocado, mashed
- Juice of 1/2 lemon

- Sprouts (such as alfalfa or broccoli sprouts)
- Salt and pepper to taste
- Red pepper flakes (optional)

Instructions:

1. Toast the slices of bread until golden and crispy.
2. In a small bowl, combine the mashed avocado and lemon juice. Mix well.
3. Spread the avocado mixture evenly on the toasted bread slices.
4. Top with sprouts and sprinkle with salt, pepper, and red pepper flakes if desired.
5. Serve immediately and enjoy the creamy and refreshing avocado toast.

Buckwheat Pancakes with Sugar-Free Berry Compote

Ingredients:

For the pancakes:

- 1 cup buckwheat flour
- 1/4 cup almond flour

- 1 tablespoon ground flaxseed mixed with 3
  tablespoons water (flax egg)
- 1 cup unsweetened almond milk
- 1 tablespoon maple syrup (optional)
- 1 teaspoon baking powder
- 1/2 teaspoon vanilla extract
- Pinch of salt

For the berry compote:
- 1 cup mixed berries (such as blueberries,
  strawberries, and blackberries)
- 1 tablespoon chia seeds
- 1 tablespoon water
- 1/2 teaspoon lemon juice

Instructions:

For the pancakes:
1. In a large mixing bowl, combine buckwheat flour,
   almond flour, baking powder, and salt.
2. In a separate bowl, whisk together the flaxseed
   mixture, almond milk, maple syrup, and vanilla
   extract.

3. Pour the wet ingredients into the dry ingredients and stir until well combined. Let the batter rest for 5-10 minutes.

4. Heat a non-stick skillet or griddle over medium heat and lightly grease with oil or cooking spray.

5. Pour 1/4 cup of batter onto the skillet for each pancake. Cook until bubbles form on the surface, then flip and cook for another 1-2 minutes until golden brown.

6. Repeat with the remaining batter. Keep the cooked pancakes warm while preparing the berry compote.

For the berry compote:

1. In a small saucepan, combine the mixed berries, chia seeds, water, and lemon juice.

2. Cook over low heat for 5-7 minutes, stirring occasionally until the berries soften and release their juices.

3. Remove from heat and let the compote cool and thicken for a few minutes.

4. Serve the buckwheat pancakes with a generous dollop of sugar-free berry compote on top.

Chia Pudding with Coconut Milk and Mango

Ingredients:

- 1/4 cup chia seeds
- 1 cup unsweetened coconut milk
- 1 tablespoon maple syrup (optional)
- 1/2 teaspoon vanilla extract
- 1 ripe mango, diced
- Shredded coconut, for garnish

Instructions:

1. In a bowl, combine chia seeds, coconut milk, maple syrup, and vanilla extract. Stir well to combine.
2. Let the mixture sit for 5 minutes, then stir again to prevent clumping of the chia seeds.
3. Cover the bowl and refrigerate for at least 2 hours or overnight to allow the chia seeds to absorb the liquid and form a pudding-like consistency.
4. Once the chia pudding has set, stir it well to break up any clumps.
5. Spoon the chia pudding into serving bowls and top with diced mango.

6. Sprinkle shredded coconut on top for added texture and flavor.

7. Enjoy the refreshing and creamy chia pudding as a delightful breakfast or snack.

Lentil and Vegetable Breakfast Bowl

Ingredients:

- 1/2 cup cooked lentils
- 1/4 cup diced cucumber
- 1/4 cup diced cherry tomatoes
- 1/4 cup diced bell peppers
- 2 tablespoons diced red onion
- 2 tablespoons chopped fresh parsley
- Juice of 1/2 lemon
- 1 tablespoon extra-virgin olive oil
- Salt and pepper to taste
- Sprouts, for garnish

Instructions:

1. In a bowl, combine cooked lentils, cucumber, cherry tomatoes, bell peppers, red onion, and parsley.

2. In a separate small bowl, whisk together lemon
    juice, olive oil, salt, and pepper.

3. Pour the dressing over the lentil and vegetable
    mixture. Toss gently to coat all the ingredients.

4. Let the flavors marinate for a few minutes.

5. Garnish the lentil and vegetable breakfast bowl with
    sprouts.

6. Serve and savor the fresh and wholesome flavors.

Green Smoothie with Spinach, Kale, and Apple

Ingredients:

- 1 cup spinach leaves
- 1 cup kale leaves
- 1 green apple, cored and chopped
- 1/2 cup unsweetened almond milk
- 1/2 cup coconut water
- 1 tablespoon almond butter
- 1 tablespoon chia seeds
- 1 teaspoon maple syrup (optional)
- Ice cubes (optional)

Instructions:

1. Place spinach leaves, kale leaves, green apple, almond milk, coconut water, almond butter, chia seeds, and maple syrup in a blender.
2. Blend on high speed until smooth and creamy.
3. If desired, add a few ice cubes to the blender and blend again until the smoothie is chilled.
4. Pour the green smoothie into glasses and serve immediately. Enjoy the refreshing and nutrient-packed drink.

Chickpea Flour Omelet with Sautéed Vegetables

Ingredients:

For the omelet:

- 1/2 cup chickpea flour
- 1/2 cup water
- 2 tablespoons nutritional yeast
- 1/2 teaspoon turmeric
- 1/4 teaspoon garlic powder
- 1/4 teaspoon onion powder
- Salt and pepper to taste

For the sautéed vegetables:

- 1 teaspoon olive oil
- 1/4 cup diced bell peppers
- 1/4 cup diced zucchini
- 1/4 cup sliced mushrooms
- 1/4 cup diced tomatoes
- Handful of spinach leaves

Instructions:

For the omelet:

1. In a bowl, whisk together chickpea flour, water, nutritional yeast, turmeric, garlic powder, onion powder, salt, and pepper until smooth.
2. Let the batter rest for 10 minutes to allow the flavors to meld.
3. Heat a non-stick skillet over medium heat and lightly grease with olive oil or cooking spray.
4. Pour the batter onto the skillet and spread it evenly to form a thin omelet.
5. Cook for 3-4 minutes, or until the edges are set and the bottom is golden brown.

6. Carefully flip the omelet using a spatula and cook for an additional 2-3 minutes on the other side.

7. Transfer the cooked omelet to a plate.

For the sautéed vegetables:
1. Heat olive oil in a skillet over medium heat.
2. Add bell peppers, zucchini, mushrooms, tomatoes, and spinach to the skillet.
3. Sauté for 5-7 minutes, or until the vegetables are tender and lightly browned.
4. Remove from heat.

To assemble:
1. Place the sautéed vegetables on one half of the omelet.
2. Gently fold the other half of the omelet over the vegetables to create a half-moon shape.
3. Transfer the omelet to a serving plate.
4. Slice into wedges and serve hot. Enjoy the savory and protein-rich chickpea flour omelet.

Overnight Oats with Almond Milk and Cinnamon

Ingredients:

- 1/2 cup rolled oats
- 1/2 cup unsweetened almond milk
- 1 tablespoon chia seeds
- 1 tablespoon maple syrup (optional)
- 1/2 teaspoon vanilla extract
- 1/2 teaspoon ground cinnamon
- 1/4 cup mixed berries (such as blueberries, raspberries, and strawberries)
- 1 tablespoon sliced almonds

Instructions:

1. In a jar or container, combine rolled oats, almond milk, chia seeds, maple syrup, vanilla extract, and ground cinnamon. Stir well to combine.
2. Cover the jar and refrigerate overnight, or for at least 4 hours, to allow the oats and chia seeds to absorb the liquid.
3. In the morning, give the overnight oats a good stir.
4. Top with mixed berries and sliced almonds.

5. Enjoy the creamy and satisfying overnight oats as a quick and nutritious breakfast option.

Sweet Potato Hash Browns with Tofu Bacon

Ingredients:

For the hash browns:

- 1 large sweet potato, grated
- 1/4 cup diced onion
- 2 tablespoons chickpea flour
- 1/2 teaspoon paprika
- 1/2 teaspoon garlic powder
- Salt and pepper to taste
- Olive oil for frying

For the tofu bacon:

- 1/2 block firm tofu, sliced into thin strips
- 2 tablespoons soy sauce or tamari
- 1 tablespoon maple syrup
- 1/2 teaspoon liquid smoke
- 1/4 teaspoon smoked paprika
- 1/4 teaspoon garlic powder

- Olive oil for frying

Instructions:

For the hash browns:

1. Place the grated sweet potato in a clean kitchen towel and squeeze out any excess moisture.
2. In a bowl, combine the grated sweet potato, diced onion, chickpea flour, paprika, garlic powder, salt, and pepper. Mix well to form a sticky mixture.
3. Heat a non-stick skillet over medium heat and add a thin layer of olive oil.
4. Take a small handful of the sweet potato mixture and shape it into a patty. Place it onto the skillet and flatten it with a spatula.
5. Cook for 3-4 minutes on each side, or until the hash browns are crispy and golden brown.
6. Repeat with the remaining sweet potato mixture. Keep the cooked hash browns warm while preparing the tofu bacon.

For the tofu bacon:

1. In a shallow dish, whisk together soy sauce or tamari, maple syrup, liquid smoke, smoked paprika, and garlic powder.
2. Place the tofu strips in the marinade, ensuring they are well coated. Let them marinate for at least 10 minutes.
3. Heat a skillet over medium heat and add a drizzle of olive oil.
4. Add the marinated tofu strips to the skillet, reserving the marinade for later use.
5. Cook the tofu strips for 3-4 minutes on each side until they are crispy and browned.
6. Pour the reserved marinade into the skillet and cook for an additional 1-2 minutes until the sauce thickens and coats the tofu.
7. Remove the tofu bacon from the skillet and set aside.

To serve:

1. Arrange the sweet potato hash browns on a plate.
2. Top with tofu bacon strips.

3. Serve hot and enjoy the delightful combination of flavors and textures.

Vegan Banana Bread with Walnuts

Ingredients:

- 2 ripe bananas, mashed
- 1/4 cup coconut oil, melted
- 1/4 cup maple syrup
- 1 teaspoon vanilla extract
- 1 cup whole wheat flour
- 1/2 cup almond flour
- 1/4 cup rolled oats
- 1 teaspoon baking powder
- 1/2 teaspoon baking soda
- 1/2 teaspoon ground cinnamon
- 1/4 teaspoon salt
- 1/2 cup chopped walnuts

Instructions:

1. Preheat the oven to 350°F (175°C). Grease a loaf pan with oil or cooking spray.

2. In a large bowl, combine mashed bananas, melted coconut oil, maple syrup, and vanilla extract. Mix well.

3. In a separate bowl, whisk together whole wheat flour, almond flour, rolled oats, baking powder, baking soda, ground cinnamon, and salt.

4. Add the dry ingredients to the wet ingredients and stir until just combined.

5. Fold in the chopped walnuts.

6. Pour the batter into the greased loaf pan and smooth the top with a spatula.

7. Bake for 45-50 minutes, or until a toothpick inserted into the center comes out clean.

8. Remove from the oven and let the banana bread cool in the pan for 10 minutes.

9. Transfer the bread to a wire rack and allow it to cool completely before slicing.

10. Slice and serve the delicious vegan banana bread as a delightful breakfast treat or snack.

Spinach and Mushroom Breakfast Burrito

Ingredients:

- 1 teaspoon olive oil
- 1/4 cup diced onion
- 1/4 cup sliced mushrooms
- 1 cup fresh spinach leaves
- 2 tablespoons nutritional yeast
- Salt and pepper to taste
- 2 whole wheat tortillas
- Salsa or hot sauce for serving (optional)

Instructions:

1. Heat olive oil in a skillet over medium heat.
2. Add diced onion and sliced mushrooms to the skillet. Sauté for 3-4 minutes, or until the vegetables are tender.
3. Add fresh spinach leaves to the skillet and cook until wilted.
4. Stir in nutritional yeast, salt, and pepper. Mix well to combine.

5. Warm the whole wheat tortillas in a separate skillet or in the microwave.

6. Spoon the spinach and mushroom filling onto each tortilla.

7. Fold the sides of the tortilla inward, then roll it up tightly to form a burrito.

8. Serve the breakfast burrito as is or with salsa or hot sauce for added flavor.

Quinoa and Vegetable Breakfast Muffins

Ingredients:

- 1 cup cooked quinoa
- 1/4 cup diced bell peppers
- 1/4 cup diced zucchini
- 1/4 cup diced cherry tomatoes
- 2 tablespoons chopped fresh parsley
- 2 tablespoons nutritional yeast
- 2 tablespoons chickpea flour
- 1/4 teaspoon garlic powder
- 1/4 teaspoon onion powder
- Salt and pepper to taste

Instructions:

1. Preheat the oven to 350°F (175°C). Grease a muffin tin with oil or cooking spray.

2. In a large bowl, combine cooked quinoa, diced bell peppers, diced zucchini, diced cherry tomatoes, chopped parsley, nutritional yeast, chickpea flour, garlic powder, onion powder, salt, and pepper. Mix well to combine.

3. Spoon the quinoa and vegetable mixture into the greased muffin tin, filling each cavity.

4. Bake for 20-25 minutes, or until the muffins are set and lightly golden.

5. Remove from the oven and let the muffins cool in the tin for 10 minutes.

6. Carefully remove the muffins from the tin and let them cool completely on a wire rack.

7. Enjoy these savory quinoa and vegetable breakfast muffins as a grab-and-go option or as part of a wholesome breakfast.

Chapter 3: Lunch Recipes

Enjoy these flavorful and nutritious lunch recipes from the Vegan Diabetic Renal Diet Cookbook!

Lentil and Vegetable Soup

Ingredients:

- 1 cup green lentils
- 4 cups vegetable broth
- 1 onion, diced
- 2 carrots, diced
- 2 celery stalks, diced
- 2 garlic cloves, minced
- 1 teaspoon cumin
- 1 teaspoon paprika
- 1 bay leaf
- Salt and pepper to taste
- Fresh parsley, chopped (for garnish)

Instructions:

1. Rinse the lentils thoroughly and set them aside.

2. In a large pot, heat some olive oil over medium heat. Add the diced onion, carrots, and celery. Sauté until the vegetables soften.

3. Add the minced garlic, cumin, paprika, and bay leaf to the pot. Stir well to coat the vegetables with the spices.

4. Pour in the vegetable broth and add the rinsed lentils. Bring the mixture to a boil.

5. Reduce the heat to low and simmer the soup for about 30 minutes or until the lentils are tender.

6. Season with salt and pepper to taste.

7. Remove the bay leaf from the soup.

8. Serve hot, garnished with fresh parsley.

Mexican Quinoa Salad with Lime Dressing

Ingredients:

- 1 cup cooked quinoa
- 1 can black beans, rinsed and drained
- 1 cup corn kernels
- 1 bell pepper, diced

- 1 cup cherry tomatoes, halved
- 1/4 cup red onion, finely chopped
- 1/4 cup fresh cilantro, chopped
- Juice of 2 limes
- 2 tablespoons olive oil
- 1 teaspoon cumin
- Salt and pepper to taste
- Avocado slices (for serving, optional)

Instructions:

1. In a large bowl, combine the cooked quinoa, black beans, corn kernels, bell pepper, cherry tomatoes, red onion, and cilantro.
2. In a separate small bowl, whisk together the lime juice, olive oil, cumin, salt, and pepper to make the dressing.
3. Pour the dressing over the quinoa mixture and toss until well combined.
4. Let the salad sit for about 15 minutes to allow the flavors to meld.
5. Serve chilled, with avocado slices on top if desired.

Chickpea and Vegetable Stir-Fry

Ingredients:

- 1 can chickpeas, rinsed and drained
- 2 cups mixed vegetables (broccoli, bell peppers, carrots, snow peas, etc.), chopped
- 1 tablespoon olive oil
- 2 garlic cloves, minced
- 1 teaspoon ginger, grated
- 2 tablespoons low-sodium soy sauce
- 1 tablespoon maple syrup
- 1 tablespoon rice vinegar
- 1/2 teaspoon sesame oil
- Sesame seeds (for garnish)

Instructions:

1. Heat the olive oil in a large skillet or wok over medium-high heat.
2. Add the minced garlic and grated ginger to the skillet and sauté for about 1 minute until fragrant.
3. Add the mixed vegetables to the skillet and stir-fry for 4-5 minutes until they are crisp-tender.

4. In a small bowl, whisk together the soy sauce,
    maple syrup, rice vinegar, and sesame oil to make
    the sauce.

5. Pour the sauce over the vegetables in the skillet and
    add the chickpeas. Stir well to coat everything
    evenly.

6. Continue cooking for another 2-3 minutes until the
    chickpeas are heated through.

7. Remove from heat and garnish with sesame seeds.

8. Serve the stir-fry over cooked rice or noodles.

Kale and White Bean Salad with Lemon Vinaigrette

Ingredients:

- 4 cups kale, destemmed and finely chopped
- 1 can white beans, rinsed and drained
- 1/4 cup red onion, thinly sliced
- 1/4 cup sun-dried tomatoes, chopped
- 2 tablespoons fresh parsley, chopped
- Juice of 1 lemon
- 2 tablespoons extra-virgin olive oil

- 1 garlic clove, minced

- Salt and pepper to taste

Instructions:

1. In a large bowl, combine the chopped kale, white beans, red onion, sun-dried tomatoes, and fresh parsley.

2. In a separate small bowl, whisk together the lemon juice, olive oil, minced garlic, salt, and pepper to make the vinaigrette.

3. Pour the vinaigrette over the kale mixture and toss well to coat.

4. Allow the salad to sit for about 10 minutes to let the flavors meld and the kale to soften slightly.

5. Serve at room temperature or chilled.

Roasted Vegetable Wrap with Hummus

Ingredients:

- 1 cup mixed vegetables (zucchini, bell peppers, eggplant, etc.), sliced

- 1 tablespoon olive oil
- Salt and pepper to taste
- 4 whole wheat tortillas
- 1/2 cup hummus
- Handful of fresh spinach leaves
- Sliced avocado (optional)

Instructions:

1. Preheat the oven to 400°F (200°C).
2. Toss the mixed vegetables with olive oil, salt, and pepper on a baking sheet.
3. Roast the vegetables in the preheated oven for 15-20 minutes until they are tender and slightly charred.
4. Warm the whole wheat tortillas in a dry skillet or microwave.
5. Spread a generous amount of hummus onto each tortilla.
6. Layer the roasted vegetables, fresh spinach leaves, and sliced avocado (if using) on top of the hummus.
7. Roll up the tortillas tightly and slice them in half.

8. Serve the roasted vegetable wraps as a nutritious
    and filling lunch option.

Sweet Potato and Black Bean Chili

Ingredients:

- 2 sweet potatoes, peeled and diced
- 1 tablespoon olive oil
- 1 onion, diced
- 2 garlic cloves, minced
- 1 red bell pepper, diced
- 1 can black beans, rinsed and drained
- 1 can diced tomatoes
- 2 cups vegetable broth
- 1 tablespoon chili powder
- 1 teaspoon cumin
- 1/2 teaspoon paprika
- Salt and pepper to taste
- Fresh cilantro, chopped (for garnish)

Instructions:

1. Heat the olive oil in a large pot over medium heat.

2. Add the diced onion, minced garlic, and diced red bell pepper to the pot. Sauté until the vegetables soften.

3. Add the diced sweet potatoes, black beans, diced tomatoes, vegetable broth, chili powder, cumin, paprika, salt, and pepper to the pot. Stir well to combine.

4. Bring the mixture to a boil, then reduce the heat to low and simmer for about 30 minutes until the sweet potatoes are tender.

5. Adjust the seasoning if needed.

6. Serve the sweet potato and black bean chili hot, garnished with fresh cilantro.

Mediterranean Stuffed Bell Peppers

Ingredients:

- 4 bell peppers (any color)
- 1 cup cooked quinoa
- 1 cup canned chickpeas, rinsed and drained
- 1/2 cup cherry tomatoes, halved
- 1/2 cup chopped cucumber
- 1/4 cup chopped Kalamata olives

- 1/4 cup crumbled vegan feta cheese

- 2 tablespoons chopped fresh parsley

- 2 tablespoons extra virgin olive oil

- 1 tablespoon lemon juice

- 1 teaspoon dried oregano

- Salt and pepper to taste

Instructions:

1. Preheat the oven to 375°F (190°C).

2. Cut the tops off the bell peppers and remove the seeds and membranes.

3. In a large mixing bowl, combine quinoa, chickpeas, cherry tomatoes, cucumber, Kalamata olives, vegan feta cheese, parsley, olive oil, lemon juice, dried oregano, salt, and pepper. Mix well.

4. Stuff each bell pepper with the quinoa mixture and place them in a baking dish.

5. Bake for 25-30 minutes or until the bell peppers are tender and slightly charred.

6. Remove from the oven and let cool for a few minutes before serving.

7. Garnish with additional chopped parsley if desired. Serve warm.

Vegan Sushi Rolls with Quinoa and Avocado

Ingredients:

- 4 nori seaweed sheets
- 2 cups cooked quinoa, cooled
- 1 ripe avocado, sliced
- 1/2 cup shredded carrots
- 1/2 cup cucumber strips
- 1/4 cup pickled ginger
- 1/4 cup soy sauce or tamari
- Wasabi and/or sriracha for serving (optional)

Instructions:

1. Place a nori seaweed sheet on a sushi mat or a clean kitchen towel.
2. Spread a thin layer of quinoa evenly over the nori sheet, leaving a small border at the top.

3. Place avocado slices, shredded carrots, cucumber strips, and pickled ginger in a line along the center of the quinoa.

4. Carefully roll the nori sheet tightly, using the sushi mat or kitchen towel to help.

5. Wet the border of the nori sheet with a little water to seal the roll.

6. Repeat the process with the remaining nori sheets and fillings.

7. Slice each sushi roll into bite-sized pieces.

8. Serve with soy sauce or tamari for dipping, and wasabi and/or sriracha for additional heat if desired.

Spinach and Lentil Salad with Balsamic Dressing

Ingredients:

- 2 cups cooked lentils, cooled
- 4 cups fresh spinach leaves
- 1 cup cherry tomatoes, halved
- 1/2 cup sliced red onion
- 1/4 cup chopped fresh basil
- 1/4 cup chopped walnuts

- 2 tablespoons balsamic vinegar
- 2 tablespoons extra virgin olive oil
- 1 teaspoon Dijon mustard
- Salt and pepper to taste

Instructions:

1. In a large mixing bowl, combine cooked lentils, spinach leaves, cherry tomatoes, red onion, basil, and walnuts.
2. In a separate small bowl, whisk together balsamic vinegar, olive oil, Dijon mustard, salt, and pepper to make the dressing.
3. Pour the dressing over the salad and toss to coat evenly.
4. Let the salad sit for a few minutes to allow the flavors to meld.
5. Serve the spinach and lentil salad as a refreshing and nutritious lunch option.

Mushroom and Barley Soup

Ingredients:

- 1 tablespoon olive oil

- 1 onion, diced
- 2 garlic cloves, minced
- 8 ounces mushrooms, sliced
- 1 carrot, diced
- 1 celery stalk, diced
- 1/2 cup pearl barley
- 4 cups vegetable broth
- 2 cups water
- 1 teaspoon dried thyme
- Salt and pepper to taste
- Fresh parsley for garnish

Instructions:

1. Heat the olive oil in a large pot over medium heat.
2. Add the onion and garlic to the pot and sauté until fragrant and softened.
3. Add the mushrooms, carrot, and celery to the pot and cook for a few more minutes until the vegetables start to soften.
4. Stir in the pearl barley, vegetable broth, water, dried thyme, salt, and pepper.

5. Bring the soup to a boil, then reduce the heat to low and cover the pot.

6. Simmer for about 45 minutes or until the barley is tender.

7. Adjust the seasoning if needed.

8. Serve the mushroom and barley soup hot, garnished with fresh parsley.

Curried Chickpea Salad Wraps

Ingredients:

- 2 cups cooked chickpeas, rinsed and drained
- 1/2 cup diced red bell pepper
- 1/2 cup diced cucumber
- 1/4 cup chopped fresh cilantro
- 1/4 cup vegan mayonnaise
- 1 tablespoon lemon juice
- 2 teaspoons curry powder
- Salt and pepper to taste
- Whole wheat wraps or lettuce leaves for serving

Instructions:

1. In a mixing bowl, combine chickpeas, red bell pepper, cucumber, cilantro, vegan mayonnaise, lemon juice, curry powder, salt, and pepper.
2. Mash the chickpeas slightly with a fork or potato masher to create a chunky texture.
3. Stir all the ingredients until well combined.
4. Taste and adjust the seasoning if desired.
5. Spread the curried chickpea salad onto whole wheat wraps or lettuce leaves.
6. Roll up the wraps tightly and secure with toothpicks if necessary.
7. Serve the curried chickpea salad wraps as a satisfying and flavorful lunch option.

Quinoa and Black Bean Burgers

Ingredients:

- 1 cup cooked quinoa, cooled
- 1 can black beans, rinsed and drained
- 1/2 cup finely chopped onion
- 1/2 cup grated carrot
- 1/4 cup chopped fresh parsley
- 1/4 cup bread crumbs (gluten-free if desired)

- 2 tablespoons ground flaxseed mixed with 6 tablespoons water (flax egg)
- 2 tablespoons soy sauce or tamari
- 1 teaspoon ground cumin
- 1/2 teaspoon smoked paprika
- Salt and pepper to taste
- Burger buns and toppings of your choice

Instructions:

1. In a large mixing bowl, mash the black beans with a fork or potato masher.
2. Add the cooked quinoa, onion, grated carrot, parsley, bread crumbs, flax egg, soy sauce, ground cumin, smoked paprika, salt, and pepper to the bowl.
3. Mix all the ingredients until well combined and the mixture holds together.
4. Shape the mixture into burger patties.
5. Heat a non-stick skillet over medium heat and lightly grease it.

6. Cook the quinoa and black bean burgers for about 4-5 minutes on each side, or until golden brown and heated through.

7. Serve the burgers on buns with your favorite toppings, such as lettuce, tomato, avocado, and condiments.

Cauliflower Fried Rice

Ingredients:

- 4 cups cauliflower rice (fresh or frozen)
- 1 cup frozen mixed vegetables
- 1/2 cup diced bell peppers
- 1/2 cup diced carrots
- 1/2 cup chopped green onions
- 3 cloves garlic, minced
- 2 tablespoons soy sauce or tamari
- 2 tablespoons sesame oil
- 1 tablespoon rice vinegar
- 1 teaspoon grated ginger
- 1/4 cup chopped fresh cilantro (optional)
- Sesame seeds for garnish (optional)

Instructions:

1. Heat the sesame oil in a large skillet or wok over medium heat.
2. Add the garlic and grated ginger to the skillet and sauté until fragrant.
3. Add the bell peppers, carrots, and frozen mixed vegetables to the skillet. Stir-fry for a few minutes until the vegetables start to soften.
4. Push the vegetables to one side of the skillet and add the cauliflower rice to the empty side. Cook for a few minutes until the cauliflower rice is heated through.
5. Stir everything together in the skillet, then add soy sauce or tamari and rice vinegar. Mix well to coat the ingredients.
6. Cook for another 2-3 minutes, stirring frequently.
7. Remove from heat and stir in the chopped green onions and fresh cilantro if using.
8. Garnish with sesame seeds if desired.
9. Serve the cauliflower fried rice as a delicious and low-carb lunch option.

Chapter 4: Dinner Recipes

In this chapter, you will discover a variety of delicious and nutritious dinner recipes that are suitable for a vegan, diabetic, and renal-friendly diet. These recipes feature wholesome ingredients and flavorful combinations to satisfy your taste buds while promoting good health.

Baked Tofu with Roasted Vegetables

Ingredients:

- 1 block of firm tofu, pressed and drained
- 2 tablespoons soy sauce
- 1 tablespoon maple syrup
- 1 tablespoon rice vinegar
- 1 teaspoon minced ginger
- 1 teaspoon minced garlic
- 1 red bell pepper, sliced
- 1 zucchini, sliced
- 1 cup cherry tomatoes
- 1 tablespoon olive oil

- Salt and pepper to taste

- Fresh cilantro for garnish

Instructions:

1. Preheat the oven to 400°F (200°C).

2. In a small bowl, whisk together the soy sauce, maple syrup, rice vinegar, minced ginger, and minced garlic.

3. Cut the tofu into cubes and place them in a baking dish. Pour the marinade over the tofu, making sure each piece is coated. Let it marinate for about 15 minutes.

4. In a separate baking dish, toss the sliced bell pepper, zucchini, and cherry tomatoes with olive oil, salt, and pepper.

5. Place both baking dishes in the preheated oven. Bake the tofu for 20-25 minutes, or until golden brown and crispy. Roast the vegetables for 15-20 minutes, or until tender.

6. Serve the baked tofu alongside the roasted vegetables. Garnish with fresh cilantro.

Spaghetti Squash with Tomato Basil Sauce

Ingredients:

- 1 medium spaghetti squash
- 2 tablespoons olive oil
- 1 small onion, finely chopped
- 2 cloves garlic, minced
- 1 can (14 ounces) diced tomatoes
- 1 tablespoon tomato paste
- 1 teaspoon dried basil
- 1 teaspoon dried oregano
- Salt and pepper to taste
- Fresh basil leaves for garnish

Instructions:

1. Preheat the oven to 400°F (200°C).
2. Cut the spaghetti squash in half lengthwise. Scoop out the seeds and discard them.
3. Brush the inside of the squash with olive oil and place both halves on a baking sheet, cut side down.

4. Bake the spaghetti squash for 40-45 minutes, or until the flesh is tender and can easily be scraped into strands with a fork.

5. While the squash is baking, heat the remaining olive oil in a saucepan over medium heat. Add the chopped onion and minced garlic, and sauté until translucent and fragrant.

6. Stir in the diced tomatoes, tomato paste, dried basil, dried oregano, salt, and pepper. Simmer the sauce for 15-20 minutes, allowing the flavors to meld together.

7. Once the spaghetti squash is cooked, use a fork to scrape the flesh into strands.

8. Serve the spaghetti squash topped with the tomato basil sauce. Garnish with fresh basil leaves.

Vegan Pad Thai with Tofu and Vegetables

Ingredients:

- 8 ounces rice noodles
- 2 tablespoons vegetable oil

- 1 block of firm tofu, pressed and cut into small cubes
- 2 cloves garlic, minced
- 1 small onion, thinly sliced
- 1 cup shredded carrots
- 1 cup bean sprouts
- 1/2 cup chopped scallions
- 1/4 cup chopped roasted peanuts
- Lime wedges for serving

Sauce:
- 2 tablespoons tamari or soy sauce
- 2 tablespoons maple syrup
- 2 tablespoons rice vinegar
- 2 tablespoons lime juice
- 1 tablespoon tamarind paste (optional)
- 1 teaspoon sriracha or chili sauce (optional)

Instructions:
1. Cook the rice noodles according to the package instructions. Drain and set aside.

2. In a small bowl, whisk together the tamari or soy sauce, maple syrup, rice vinegar, lime juice, tamarind paste (if using), and sriracha or chili sauce (if using). Set the sauce aside.

3. Heat the vegetable oil in a large skillet or wok over medium-high heat. Add the tofu cubes and cook until golden brown and crispy. Remove the tofu from the skillet and set aside.

4. In the same skillet, add the minced garlic, sliced onion, and shredded carrots. Stir-fry for a few minutes until the vegetables are slightly softened.

5. Add the cooked rice noodles, bean sprouts, and the prepared sauce to the skillet. Toss everything together until well coated and heated through.

6. Stir in the cooked tofu and chopped scallions. Cook for an additional minute to combine the flavors.

7. Remove from heat and garnish with chopped roasted peanuts.

8. Serve the vegan Pad Thai with lime wedges for squeezing fresh lime juice over the dish.

Stuffed Portobello Mushrooms with Quinoa and Spinach

Ingredients:

- 4 large portobello mushrooms
- 1 cup cooked quinoa
- 1 cup fresh spinach, chopped
- 1 small onion, finely chopped
- 2 cloves garlic, minced
- 1/4 cup nutritional yeast
- 2 tablespoons chopped fresh basil
- 2 tablespoons olive oil
- Salt and pepper to taste

Instructions:

1. Preheat the oven to 375°F (190°C).
2. Remove the stems from the portobello mushrooms and gently scrape out the gills using a spoon.
3. In a large skillet, heat the olive oil over medium heat. Add the chopped onion and minced garlic, and sauté until translucent and fragrant.
4. Add the chopped spinach to the skillet and cook until wilted.

5. In a mixing bowl, combine the cooked quinoa, sautéed spinach, nutritional yeast, chopped fresh basil, salt, and pepper. Mix well to combine.

6. Place the portobello mushrooms on a baking sheet and divide the quinoa mixture among them, stuffing it into the mushroom caps.

7. Bake the stuffed mushrooms for 20-25 minutes, or until the mushrooms are tender and the filling is heated through.

8. Serve the stuffed portobello mushrooms as a flavorful and hearty main course.

Moroccan Chickpea Stew with Couscous

Ingredients:

- 1 tablespoon olive oil
- 1 small onion, finely chopped
- 2 cloves garlic, minced
- 1 teaspoon ground cumin
- 1 teaspoon ground coriander
- 1/2 teaspoon ground cinnamon
- 1/4 teaspoon ground turmeric

- 1 can (14 ounces) diced tomatoes
- 2 cups vegetable broth
- 2 cups cooked chickpeas
- 1 cup chopped carrots
- 1 cup chopped bell peppers
- 1/2 cup dried apricots, chopped
- 1/4 cup chopped fresh parsley
- Salt and pepper to taste
- Cooked couscous for serving

Instructions:

1. Heat the olive oil in a large pot or Dutch oven over medium heat. Add the chopped onion and minced garlic, and sauté until fragrant and softened.
2. Stir in the ground cumin, ground coriander, ground cinnamon, and ground turmeric. Cook for an additional minute to toast the spices.
3. Add the diced tomatoes, vegetable broth, cooked chickpeas, chopped carrots, chopped bell peppers, and dried apricots to the pot. Stir to combine.
4. Bring the mixture to a boil, then reduce the heat to low. Cover the pot and simmer for 20-25 minutes,

or until the vegetables are tender and the flavors have melded together.

5. Stir in the chopped fresh parsley and season with salt and pepper to taste.

6. Serve the Moroccan chickpea stew over cooked couscous for a hearty and satisfying dinner.

Ratatouille with Quinoa Pilaf

Ingredients:

Ratatouille:

- 2 tablespoons olive oil
- 1 small onion, diced
- 2 cloves garlic, minced
- 1 small eggplant, diced
- 1 zucchini, diced
- 1 yellow bell pepper, diced
- 1 red bell pepper, diced
- 1 can (14 ounces) diced tomatoes
- 1 tablespoon tomato paste
- 1 teaspoon dried thyme
- 1 teaspoon dried oregano
- Salt and pepper to taste

- Fresh basil leaves for garnish

Quinoa Pilaf:

- 1 cup quinoa
- 2 cups vegetable broth
- 1 tablespoon olive oil
- 1 small onion, finely chopped
- 1 carrot, finely chopped
- 1 celery stalk, finely chopped
- 1/4 cup chopped fresh parsley
- Salt and pepper to taste

Instructions:

1. Heat the olive oil in a large pot or Dutch oven over medium heat. Add the diced onion and minced garlic, and sauté until translucent and fragrant.

2. Add the diced eggplant, diced zucchini, diced yellow and red bell peppers to the pot. Sauté the vegetables for a few minutes until slightly softened.

3. Stir in the diced tomatoes, tomato paste, dried thyme, dried oregano, salt, and pepper. Cover the pot and simmer for 20-25 minutes, or until the

vegetables are tender and the flavors have melded together.

4. Meanwhile, prepare the quinoa pilaf. Rinse the quinoa under cold water.

5. In a saucepan, heat the olive oil over medium heat. Add the finely chopped onion, carrot, and celery. Sauté until the vegetables are softened.

6. Add the rinsed quinoa to the saucepan and stir to combine with the sautéed vegetables.

7. Pour in the vegetable broth and bring the mixture to a boil. Reduce the heat to low, cover the saucepan, and simmer for 15-20 minutes, or until the quinoa is cooked and the liquid has been absorbed.

8. Fluff the quinoa pilaf with a fork and stir in the chopped fresh parsley. Season with salt and pepper to taste.

9. Serve the ratatouille with quinoa pilaf, garnished with fresh basil leaves.

Vegan Lentil Loaf with Mashed Cauliflower

Ingredients:

Lentil Loaf:

- 1 cup green or brown lentils, cooked
- 1 small onion, finely chopped
- 2 cloves garlic, minced
- 1 carrot, grated
- 1 celery stalk, finely chopped
- 1/2 cup rolled oats
- 1/4 cup nutritional yeast
- 2 tablespoons tomato paste
- 2 tablespoons soy sauce
- 1 tablespoon ground flaxseeds mixed with 3 tablespoons water (flax egg)
- 1 teaspoon dried thyme
- 1/2 teaspoon dried rosemary
- Salt and pepper to taste

Mashed Cauliflower:

- 1 medium head of cauliflower, cut into florets
- 2 cloves garlic
- 2 tablespoons vegan butter or olive oil
- Salt and pepper to taste
- Chopped fresh parsley for garnish

Instructions:

1. Preheat the oven to 375°F (190°C). Grease a loaf pan and set aside.

2. In a large bowl, combine the cooked lentils, finely chopped onion, minced garlic, grated carrot, finely chopped celery, rolled oats, nutritional yeast, tomato paste, soy sauce, flax egg, dried thyme, dried rosemary, salt, and pepper. Mix well until all the ingredients are evenly distributed.

3. Transfer the lentil mixture into the greased loaf pan and press it down firmly.

4. Bake the lentil loaf in the preheated oven for 40-45 minutes, or until the top is firm and golden brown.

5. While the lentil loaf is baking, prepare the mashed cauliflower. Steam or boil the cauliflower florets and garlic cloves until they are soft and easily mashed.

6. Drain the cooked cauliflower and garlic. Transfer them to a bowl and mash them with a potato masher or blend them in a food processor until smooth.

7. Stir in the vegan butter or olive oil, salt, and pepper. Adjust the seasoning to your taste.

8. Once the lentil loaf is cooked, remove it from the oven and let it cool for a few minutes before slicing.

9. Serve slices of the lentil loaf with a generous dollop of mashed cauliflower. Garnish with chopped fresh parsley.

Coconut Curry with Chickpeas and Brown Rice

Ingredients:

- 1 tablespoon coconut oil
- 1 small onion, finely chopped
- 2 cloves garlic, minced
- 1 tablespoon grated fresh ginger
- 1 tablespoon curry powder
- 1 teaspoon ground turmeric
- 1 can (14 ounces) coconut milk
- 1 can (14 ounces) diced tomatoes
- 2 cups cooked chickpeas
- 1 cup chopped vegetables (e.g., bell peppers, carrots, green beans)
- 1 cup spinach leaves
- Salt and pepper to taste

- Cooked brown rice for serving
- Fresh cilantro for garnish

Instructions:

1. Heat the coconut oil in a large pot or skillet over medium heat. Add the finely chopped onion, minced garlic, and grated fresh ginger. Sauté until fragrant and the onion is translucent.
2. Stir in the curry powder and ground turmeric. Cook for an additional minute to toast the spices.
3. Pour in the coconut milk and diced tomatoes, including their juices. Stir well to combine.
4. Add the cooked chickpeas and chopped vegetables to the pot. Bring the mixture to a simmer and let it cook for about 10 minutes, or until the vegetables are tender.
5. Stir in the spinach leaves and cook for an additional minute until wilted.
6. Season the coconut curry with salt and pepper to taste.
7. Serve the coconut curry over cooked brown rice. Garnish with fresh cilantro.

Zucchini Noodles with Creamy Cashew Sauce

Ingredients:

- 4 medium zucchini
- 1 cup raw cashews, soaked in water for at least 2 hours
- 2 cloves garlic
- 2 tablespoons nutritional yeast
- 2 tablespoons lemon juice
- 1/4 cup water (or more as needed)
- Salt and pepper to taste
- Chopped fresh parsley for garnish

Instructions:

1. Trim the ends of the zucchini and spiralize them into noodles using a spiralizer or julienne peeler. Set the zucchini noodles aside.
2. Drain the soaked cashews and rinse them under cold water.
3. In a blender or food processor, combine the soaked cashews, garlic cloves, nutritional yeast, lemon juice, water, salt, and pepper. Blend until smooth

and creamy. If needed, add more water to achieve your desired consistency.

4. In a large skillet, heat a small amount of oil over medium heat. Add the zucchini noodles and sauté for 2-3 minutes until slightly softened but still crisp.

5. Pour the creamy cashew sauce over the zucchini noodles and toss to coat evenly.

6. Cook for an additional 2-3 minutes until the sauce is heated through.

7. Remove from heat and garnish with chopped fresh parsley.

8. Serve the zucchini noodles with creamy cashew sauce as a light and flavorful dinner.

Black Bean and Vegetable Enchiladas

Ingredients:

Enchilada Filling:

- 1 tablespoon olive oil
- 1 small onion, finely chopped
- 2 cloves garlic, minced
- 1 bell pepper, diced

- 1 zucchini, diced

- 1 cup corn kernels

- 1 can (14 ounces) black beans, rinsed and drained

- 1 cup diced tomatoes

- 1 teaspoon ground cumin

- 1/2 teaspoon chili powder

- Salt and pepper to taste

Enchilada Sauce:

- 1 can (14 ounces) diced tomatoes

- 1 tablespoon tomato paste

- 1 teaspoon ground cumin

- 1/2 teaspoon chili powder

- Salt and pepper to taste

Enchilada Assembly:

- 8 small tortillas (corn or flour)

- 1 cup shredded vegan cheese (optional)

- Fresh cilantro for garnish

Instructions:

1. Preheat the oven to 375°F (190°C).

2. Heat the olive oil in a large skillet over medium heat. Add the finely chopped onion, minced garlic, diced bell pepper, and diced zucchini. Sauté until the vegetables are slightly softened.

3. Stir in the corn kernels, black beans, diced tomatoes, ground cumin, chili powder, salt, and pepper. Cook for a few minutes until heated through.

4. In a blender or food processor, combine the diced tomatoes, tomato paste, ground cumin, chili powder, salt, and pepper. Blend until smooth to make the enchilada sauce.

5. Spread a thin layer of the enchilada sauce on the bottom of a baking dish.

6. Place a small amount of the vegetable and black bean filling in the center of each tortilla. Roll up the tortilla and place it seam-side down in the baking dish.

7. Repeat the process with the remaining tortillas and filling.

8. Pour the remaining enchilada sauce over the assembled enchiladas. If desired, sprinkle shredded vegan cheese on top.

9. Cover the baking dish with foil and bake in the preheated oven for 20-25 minutes, or until the enchiladas are heated through and the cheese is melted.

10. Remove from the oven and garnish with fresh cilantro.

11. Serve the black bean and vegetable enchiladas as a flavorful and satisfying dinner.

Stuffed Bell Peppers with Quinoa and Black Beans

Ingredients:

- 4 bell peppers (any color), tops removed and seeds discarded
- 1 cup cooked quinoa
- 1 can (14 ounces) black beans, rinsed and drained
- 1 small onion, finely chopped
- 2 cloves garlic, minced
- 1 cup diced tomatoes

- 1/2 cup corn kernels

- 1 teaspoon ground cumin

- 1/2 teaspoon chili powder

- Salt and pepper to taste

- Fresh cilantro for garnish

Instructions:

1. Preheat the oven to 375°F (190°C). Grease a baking dish and set aside.

2. In a large bowl, combine the cooked quinoa, rinsed black beans, finely chopped onion, minced garlic, diced tomatoes, corn kernels, ground cumin, chili powder, salt, and pepper. Mix well to combine.

3. Stuff each bell pepper with the quinoa and black bean mixture. Place the stuffed bell peppers in the greased baking dish.

4. Cover the dish with foil and bake in the preheated oven for 30-35 minutes, or until the bell peppers are tender.

5. Remove the foil and bake for an additional 5 minutes to lightly brown the tops.

6. Remove from the oven and garnish with fresh cilantro.

7. Serve the stuffed bell peppers with quinoa and black beans as a wholesome and colorful dinner.

Teriyaki Tofu Stir-Fry with Brown Rice

Ingredients:

Teriyaki Sauce:

- 1/4 cup tamari or soy sauce
- 2 tablespoons maple syrup
- 1 tablespoon rice vinegar
- 1 tablespoon cornstarch
- 1/4 cup water

Stir-Fry:

- 1 tablespoon sesame oil
- 1 block of firm tofu, pressed and cut into cubes
- 1 small onion, sliced
- 1 bell pepper, sliced
- 1 cup broccoli florets
- 1 carrot, thinly sliced

- 1 cup snap peas
- Cooked brown rice for serving
- Sesame seeds for garnish
- Chopped green onions for garnish

Instructions:

1. In a small bowl, whisk together the tamari or soy sauce, maple syrup, rice vinegar, cornstarch, and water to make the teriyaki sauce. Set the sauce aside.

2. Heat the sesame oil in a large skillet or wok over medium-high heat. Add the tofu cubes and cook until golden brown and crispy. Remove the tofu from the skillet and set aside.

3. In the same skillet, add the sliced onion, sliced bell pepper, broccoli florets, carrot slices, and snap peas. Stir-fry the vegetables until they are crisp-tender.

4. Pour the teriyaki sauce over the vegetables in the skillet. Cook for a few minutes until the sauce thickens and coats the vegetables.

5. Return the cooked tofu to the skillet and toss everything together to combine.

6. Remove from heat and serve the teriyaki tofu stir-fry over cooked brown rice.

7. Garnish with sesame seeds and chopped green onions.

Creamy Vegan Alfredo Pasta with Broccoli

Ingredients:

- 8 ounces fettuccine pasta (or pasta of your choice)
- 2 cups broccoli florets
- 1 tablespoon olive oil
- 1 small onion, finely chopped
- 2 cloves garlic, minced
- 1 cup cashews, soaked in water for at least 2 hours
- 1 cup vegetable broth
- 1 tablespoon nutritional yeast
- 1 tablespoon lemon juice
- Salt and pepper to taste
- Chopped fresh parsley for garnish

Instructions:

1. Cook the fettuccine pasta according to the package instructions. Drain and set aside.

2. Steam or boil the broccoli florets until they are tender. Drain and set aside.

3. In a large skillet, heat the olive oil over medium heat. Add the finely chopped onion and minced garlic. Sauté until fragrant and the onion is translucent.

4. Drain the soaked cashews and rinse them under cold water.

5. In a blender or food processor, combine the soaked cashews, vegetable broth, nutritional yeast, lemon juice, salt, and pepper. Blend until smooth and creamy.

6. Pour the cashew sauce into the skillet with the sautéed onion and garlic. Stir well to combine and heat the sauce until warmed through.

7. Add the cooked fettuccine pasta and steamed broccoli to the skillet. Toss everything together until the pasta and broccoli are coated with the creamy sauce.

8. Cook for an additional minute or two until everything is heated through.

9. Remove from heat and garnish with chopped fresh parsley.

10. Serve the creamy vegan Alfredo pasta with broccoli as a comforting and satisfying dinner.

Enjoy these delicious and nutritious snacks and appetizers from Chapter 5 of the Vegan Diabetic Renal Diet Cookbook!

Roasted Chickpeas with Spices

Ingredients:

- 1 can (15 ounces) chickpeas, drained and rinsed
- 1 tablespoon olive oil
- 1 teaspoon paprika
- 1/2 teaspoon ground cumin
- 1/2 teaspoon garlic powder
- 1/4 teaspoon cayenne pepper (optional)
- Salt to taste

Instructions:

1. Preheat the oven to 400°F (200°C).
2. Pat dry the chickpeas using a kitchen towel or paper towel.

3. In a bowl, toss the chickpeas with olive oil, paprika, cumin, garlic powder, cayenne pepper (if using), and salt.

4. Spread the seasoned chickpeas in a single layer on a baking sheet.

5. Roast in the preheated oven for 25-30 minutes, or until the chickpeas are crispy and golden brown.

6. Remove from the oven and let them cool before serving.

7. Enjoy as a crunchy and protein-packed snack!

Guacamole with Baked Tortilla Chips

Ingredients:

For Guacamole:

- 2 ripe avocados
- 1 small tomato, diced
- 1/4 cup red onion, finely chopped
- 1/4 cup cilantro, chopped
- 1 tablespoon lime juice
- 1 clove garlic, minced
- Salt and pepper to taste

For Baked Tortilla Chips:

- 4 corn tortillas
- Cooking spray
- Salt to taste

Instructions:

For Guacamole:

1. Cut the avocados in half, remove the pits, and scoop the flesh into a bowl.
2. Mash the avocados with a fork until desired consistency.
3. Add the diced tomato, red onion, cilantro, lime juice, minced garlic, salt, and pepper to the mashed avocados. Mix well.
4. Taste and adjust the seasonings if needed.
5. Cover the guacamole and refrigerate for at least 30 minutes to allow the flavors to meld.

For Baked Tortilla Chips:

1. Preheat the oven to 375°F (190°C).
2. Stack the corn tortillas and cut them into quarters to make triangle-shaped chips.

3. Arrange the tortilla chips in a single layer on a baking sheet lined with parchment paper.

4. Lightly spray the tortilla chips with cooking spray and sprinkle salt over them.

5. Bake in the preheated oven for 10-12 minutes, or until the chips are crispy and golden brown.

6. Remove from the oven and let them cool before serving.

7. Serve the freshly made guacamole with the baked tortilla chips for a delicious and healthy snack.

Vegan Spinach Artichoke Dip

Ingredients:

- 1 cup frozen spinach, thawed and squeezed dry
- 1 can (14 ounces) artichoke hearts, drained and chopped
- 1 cup vegan mayonnaise
- 1 cup vegan cream cheese
- 1/2 cup nutritional yeast
- 1/4 cup grated vegan Parmesan cheese
- 2 cloves garlic, minced
- 1/2 teaspoon onion powder

- 1/2 teaspoon dried dill

- Salt and pepper to taste

Instructions:

1. Preheat the oven to 350°F (175°C).
2. In a large bowl, combine the thawed and squeezed dry spinach, chopped artichoke hearts, vegan mayonnaise, vegan cream cheese, nutritional yeast, grated vegan Parmesan cheese, minced garlic, onion powder, dried dill, salt, and pepper. Mix well.
3. Transfer the mixture to an oven-safe baking dish and spread it out evenly.
4. Bake in the preheated oven for 25-30 minutes, or until the dip is hot and bubbly.
5. Remove from the oven and let it cool for a few minutes before serving.
6. Serve the vegan spinach artichoke dip with crackers, sliced baguette, or vegetable sticks.

Carrot and Hummus Sticks

Ingredients:

- 2 large carrots, peeled and cut into sticks

- 1 cup hummus (store-bought or homemade)

Instructions:

1. Wash, peel, and cut the carrots into sticks.
2. Arrange the carrot sticks on a plate or serving platter.
3. Place the hummus in a small bowl and serve it alongside the carrot sticks as a dipping sauce.
4. Dip the carrot sticks into the hummus and enjoy a healthy and flavorful snack.

Oven-Baked Sweet Potato Fries

Ingredients:

- 2 large sweet potatoes
- 2 tablespoons olive oil
- 1 teaspoon paprika
- 1/2 teaspoon garlic powder
- 1/2 teaspoon onion powder
- 1/4 teaspoon cayenne pepper (optional)
- Salt to taste

Instructions:

1. Preheat the oven to 425°F (220°C).

2. Peel the sweet potatoes and cut them into fries, about 1/4-inch thick.

3. In a large bowl, toss the sweet potato fries with olive oil, paprika, garlic powder, onion powder, cayenne pepper (if using), and salt.

4. Spread the seasoned sweet potato fries in a single layer on a baking sheet lined with parchment paper.

5. Bake in the preheated oven for 25-30 minutes, flipping halfway through, or until the fries are crispy and golden brown.

6. Remove from the oven and let them cool slightly before serving.

7. Serve the oven-baked sweet potato fries as a healthier alternative to traditional fries.

Cucumber Sushi Rolls with Avocado

Ingredients:

- 2 large cucumbers
- 1 ripe avocado, sliced
- 1/2 cup cooked sushi rice
- 2 tablespoons rice vinegar

- 2 teaspoons sugar
- 1/2 teaspoon salt
- Soy sauce for dipping
- Wasabi and pickled ginger (optional)

Instructions:

1. Peel the cucumbers and cut them into long, thin strips using a vegetable peeler or a mandoline slicer.
2. In a small bowl, combine rice vinegar, sugar, and salt. Stir until the sugar and salt dissolve.
3. Place the cucumber strips in a bowl and pour the rice vinegar mixture over them. Toss gently to coat the cucumber strips. Let them marinate for 10-15 minutes.
4. Lay a cucumber strip flat on a clean surface and place a slice of avocado and a spoonful of sushi rice at one end.
5. Carefully roll the cucumber strip, enclosing the avocado and sushi rice, until you reach the other end.
6. Repeat with the remaining cucumber strips, avocado, and sushi rice.

7. Serve the cucumber sushi rolls with soy sauce for dipping. Optionally, serve with wasabi and pickled ginger for added flavor.

Spicy Edamame

Ingredients:

- 2 cups frozen edamame, in shells
- 2 tablespoons soy sauce
- 1 tablespoon sriracha sauce
- 1 tablespoon sesame oil
- 1/2 teaspoon garlic powder
- 1/2 teaspoon ground ginger
- 1/2 teaspoon sesame seeds (optional)

Instructions:

1. Cook the edamame according to the package instructions. Drain and set aside.
2. In a small bowl, whisk together soy sauce, sriracha sauce, sesame oil, garlic powder, ground ginger, and sesame seeds (if using).

3. Heat a large skillet over medium heat. Add the cooked edamame and the sauce mixture to the skillet.

4. Stir-fry the edamame in the sauce for 2-3 minutes, or until heated through and well-coated with the sauce.

5. Remove from the heat and transfer the spicy edamame to a serving bowl.

6. Sprinkle with additional sesame seeds if desired.

7. Serve the spicy edamame as a flavorful and protein-packed snack.

Mediterranean Stuffed Grape Leaves

Ingredients:

- 1 jar (8 ounces) grape leaves, drained
- 1 cup cooked quinoa
- 1/2 cup chopped Kalamata olives
- 1/4 cup chopped sun-dried tomatoes
- 1/4 cup chopped fresh parsley
- 1/4 cup chopped fresh mint
- 2 tablespoons lemon juice
- 2 tablespoons olive oil

- Salt and pepper to taste

Instructions:

1. Rinse the grape leaves under cold water and drain.
2. In a bowl, combine cooked quinoa, chopped Kalamata olives, chopped sun-dried tomatoes, chopped fresh parsley, chopped fresh mint, lemon juice, olive oil, salt, and pepper. Mix well.
3. Lay a grape leaf flat on a clean surface and place a spoonful of the quinoa mixture near the stem end.
4. Fold the sides of the grape leaf inward and roll it tightly from the stem end to the tip, enclosing the filling.
5. Repeat with the remaining grape leaves and quinoa mixture.
6. Place the stuffed grape leaves in a serving dish.
7. Serve the Mediterranean stuffed grape leaves chilled or at room temperature as an appetizer or part of a mezze platter.

Vegan Nachos with Cashew Cheese

Ingredients:

For Cashew Cheese:

- 1 cup raw cashews, soaked in water for at least 4 hours, drained
- 1/4 cup nutritional yeast
- 2 tablespoons lemon juice
- 1 clove garlic
- 1/2 teaspoon onion powder
- 1/2 teaspoon paprika
- 1/4 teaspoon turmeric
- 1/4 teaspoon salt
- 1/4 teaspoon cayenne pepper (optional)
- Water (as needed for consistency)

For Nachos:

- 1 bag tortilla chips
- 1 cup cooked black beans, drained and rinsed
- 1/2 cup diced tomatoes
- 1/2 cup sliced black olives
- 1/4 cup chopped fresh cilantro
- Pickled jalapeños (optional)

Instructions:

For Cashew Cheese:

1. In a blender or food processor, combine soaked and drained cashews, nutritional yeast, lemon juice, garlic, onion powder, paprika, turmeric, salt, cayenne pepper (if using), and a splash of water.
2. Blend until smooth and creamy, adding more water as needed to achieve the desired consistency of cheese sauce. Set aside.

For Nachos:

1. Preheat the oven to 350°F (175°C).
2. Arrange the tortilla chips in a single layer on a large baking sheet.
3. Spoon the cooked black beans over the tortilla chips, distributing them evenly.
4. Drizzle the cashew cheese sauce over the nachos, covering them generously.
5. Sprinkle diced tomatoes, sliced black olives, and chopped fresh cilantro over the nachos.
6. Add pickled jalapeños if desired for an extra kick.

7. Bake in the preheated oven for 10-15 minutes, or until the nachos are heated through and the cheese sauce is bubbly.

8. Remove from the oven and let them cool slightly before serving.

9. Serve the vegan nachos as a crowd-pleasing and flavorful snack or appetizer.

Roasted Red Pepper and Walnut Dip

Ingredients:

- 2 large red bell peppers
- 1 cup walnuts
- 2 cloves garlic, minced
- 2 tablespoons olive oil
- 2 tablespoons lemon juice
- 1 tablespoon tomato paste
- 1 teaspoon ground cumin
- 1/2 teaspoon smoked paprika
- Salt and pepper to taste

Instructions:

1. Preheat the broiler in your oven.

2. Place the red bell peppers on a baking sheet and broil, turning occasionally, until the skin is charred and blistered on all sides.

3. Remove the peppers from the oven and transfer them to a bowl. Cover the bowl with plastic wrap and let the peppers steam for 10 minutes.

4. After steaming, remove the peppers from the bowl and peel off the charred skin. Cut off the stems and remove the seeds. Set aside.

5. In a food processor, combine the walnuts, minced garlic, olive oil, lemon juice, tomato paste, ground cumin, smoked paprika, salt, and pepper.

6. Add the roasted red peppers to the food processor and blend until the dip reaches a smooth and creamy consistency.

7. Taste and adjust the seasonings if needed.

8. Transfer the roasted red pepper and walnut dip to a serving bowl.

9. Serve the dip with crackers, toasted pita bread, or vegetable sticks for a flavorful and nutritious appetizer.

Crispy Baked Tofu Bites

Ingredients:

- 1 block (14 ounces) firm tofu, drained and pressed
- 2 tablespoons cornstarch
- 1 teaspoon garlic powder
- 1 teaspoon onion powder
- 1/2 teaspoon paprika
- 1/4 teaspoon salt
- Cooking spray

Instructions:

1. Preheat the oven to 400°F (200°C).
2. Cut the pressed tofu into bite-sized cubes.
3. In a shallow bowl, combine cornstarch, garlic powder, onion powder, paprika, and salt.
4. Toss the tofu cubes in the cornstarch mixture until evenly coated.
5. Line a baking sheet with parchment paper and arrange the coated tofu cubes in a single layer.
6. Lightly spray the tofu cubes with cooking spray.
7. Bake in the preheated oven for 20-25 minutes, or until the tofu bites are golden brown and crispy.

8. Remove from the oven and let them cool slightly before serving.

9. Serve the crispy baked tofu bites as a protein-rich and flavorful snack or appetizer.

Stuffed Mushrooms with Herbed Quinoa

Ingredients:

- 12 large button mushrooms
- 1 cup cooked quinoa
- 1/4 cup chopped red onion
- 1/4 cup chopped sun-dried tomatoes
- 2 tablespoons chopped fresh parsley
- 2 tablespoons chopped fresh basil
- 2 tablespoons nutritional yeast
- 1 tablespoon olive oil
- 1 clove garlic, minced
- Salt and pepper to taste

Instructions:

1. Preheat the oven to 375°F (190°C).

2. Remove the stems from the mushrooms and set them aside.

3. In a bowl, combine cooked quinoa, chopped red onion, chopped sun-dried tomatoes, chopped fresh parsley, chopped fresh basil, nutritional yeast, olive oil, minced garlic, salt, and pepper. Mix well.

4. Spoon the quinoa mixture into the mushroom caps, filling them generously.

5. Place the stuffed mushrooms on a baking sheet lined with parchment paper.

6. Bake in the preheated oven for 20-25 minutes, or until the mushrooms are tender and the filling is heated through.

7. Remove from the oven and let them cool slightly before serving.

8. Serve the stuffed mushrooms as an elegant and savory appetizer.

Baked Kale Chips with Sea Salt

Ingredients:

- 1 bunch kale
- 1 tablespoon olive oil

- Sea salt to taste

Instructions:

1. Preheat the oven to 300°F (150°C).
2. Wash the kale leaves and pat them dry with a kitchen towel or paper towel.
3. Remove the tough stems from the kale leaves and tear them into bite-sized pieces.
4. In a large bowl, drizzle the torn kale leaves with olive oil and sprinkle with sea salt.
5. Toss the kale leaves until they are well-coated with oil and salt.
6. Arrange the kale leaves in a single layer on a baking sheet lined with parchment paper.
7. Bake in the preheated oven for 10-15 minutes, or until the kale leaves are crispy and lightly browned.
8. Remove from the oven and let them cool before serving.
9. Serve the baked kale chips as a healthy and flavorful alternative to traditional potato chips.

Chapter 6: Desserts

Vegan Chocolate Avocado Mousse

Ingredients:

- 2 ripe avocados
- 1/4 cup unsweetened cocoa powder
- 1/4 cup maple syrup
- 1/4 cup almond milk
- 1 teaspoon vanilla extract
- Pinch of salt
- Fresh berries, for garnish (optional)

Instructions:

1. Cut the avocados in half, remove the pits, and scoop out the flesh into a blender or food processor.
2. Add the cocoa powder, maple syrup, almond milk, vanilla extract, and salt to the blender.
3. Blend until smooth and creamy, scraping down the sides as needed.
4. Transfer the mousse to serving bowls or glasses.
5. Chill in the refrigerator for at least 30 minutes to allow the flavors to meld.

6. Garnish with fresh berries, if desired, before serving.

Berry and Coconut Chia Seed Pudding

Ingredients:

- 1 cup unsweetened coconut milk
- 1/4 cup chia seeds
- 1 tablespoon maple syrup
- 1/2 teaspoon vanilla extract
- 1 cup mixed berries (such as strawberries, blueberries, and raspberries)
- Shredded coconut, for garnish (optional)

Instructions:

1. In a bowl, combine the coconut milk, chia seeds, maple syrup, and vanilla extract.
2. Stir well to make sure the chia seeds are evenly distributed.
3. Cover the bowl and refrigerate for at least 2 hours or overnight, allowing the chia seeds to absorb the liquid and thicken.

4. When ready to serve, give the pudding a good stir to break up any clumps.

5. Divide the pudding into serving glasses or bowls.

6. Top with mixed berries and shredded coconut, if desired.

7. Serve chilled.

Baked Apples with Cinnamon and Walnuts

Ingredients:

- 4 apples (such as Granny Smith or Honeycrisp)
- 2 tablespoons maple syrup
- 1 teaspoon ground cinnamon
- 1/4 cup chopped walnuts
- Vegan vanilla ice cream, for serving (optional)

Instructions:

1. Preheat the oven to 375°F (190°C).

2. Cut the apples in half horizontally and remove the cores with a spoon or apple corer.

3. Place the apple halves in a baking dish, cut side up.

4. Drizzle the maple syrup over the apples, then sprinkle with ground cinnamon.

5. Sprinkle the chopped walnuts evenly over the apples.

6. Bake for 25-30 minutes, or until the apples are tender and slightly caramelized.

7. Remove from the oven and let cool for a few minutes.

8. Serve the baked apples warm, optionally topped with a scoop of vegan vanilla ice cream.

Vegan Pumpkin Pie Bars

Ingredients:

Crust:

- 1 1/2 cups graham cracker crumbs (vegan if desired)
- 1/4 cup melted vegan butter

Filling:

- 1 can (15 ounces) pumpkin puree
- 1/2 cup coconut milk
- 1/2 cup maple syrup

- 1/4 cup cornstarch

- 1 teaspoon vanilla extract

- 1 teaspoon ground cinnamon

- 1/2 teaspoon ground ginger

- 1/4 teaspoon ground nutmeg

- 1/4 teaspoon salt

Topping:

- Vegan whipped cream, for serving (optional)

Instructions:

1. Preheat the oven to 350°F (175°C) and line a square baking dish with parchment paper.

2. In a bowl, combine the graham cracker crumbs and melted vegan butter for the crust.

3. Press the mixture into the bottom of the prepared baking dish to form an even layer.

4. In another bowl, whisk together the pumpkin puree, coconut milk, maple syrup, cornstarch, vanilla extract, ground cinnamon, ground ginger, ground nutmeg, and salt until smooth.

5. Pour the filling over the crust and spread it out evenly.

6. Bake for 40-45 minutes, or until the filling is set.

7. Remove from the oven and let cool completely in the baking dish.

8. Once cooled, cut into bars and serve with a dollop of vegan whipped cream, if desired.

Coconut Rice Pudding with Mango

Ingredients:

- 1 cup cooked white rice
- 1 can (13.5 ounces) coconut milk
- 1/4 cup maple syrup
- 1 teaspoon vanilla extract
- 1/4 teaspoon ground cardamom
- 1/4 teaspoon ground cinnamon
- 1 ripe mango, diced
- Toasted coconut flakes, for garnish (optional)

Instructions:

1. In a saucepan, combine the cooked white rice, coconut milk, maple syrup, vanilla extract, ground cardamom, and ground cinnamon.

2. Bring the mixture to a simmer over medium heat, stirring occasionally.

3. Reduce the heat to low and let the pudding simmer for 15-20 minutes, or until it thickens to your desired consistency, stirring occasionally.

4. Remove the pudding from the heat and let it cool for a few minutes.

5. Divide the pudding into serving bowls or glasses.

6. Top with diced mango and sprinkle with toasted coconut flakes, if desired.

7. Serve warm or chilled.

Vegan Banana Ice Cream with Peanut Butter

Ingredients:

- 4 ripe bananas, sliced and frozen
- 2 tablespoons peanut butter
- 2 tablespoons maple syrup
- Crushed peanuts, for garnish (optional)

Instructions:

1. Place the frozen banana slices, peanut butter, and maple syrup in a blender or food processor.
2. Blend until smooth and creamy, scraping down the sides as needed.
3. Transfer the banana ice cream to a freezer-safe container and freeze for about 1 hour to firm up.
4. When ready to serve, scoop the banana ice cream into bowls or cones.
5. Garnish with crushed peanuts, if desired.
6. Enjoy immediately.

Lemon Poppy Seed Energy Balls

Ingredients:

- 1 cup pitted dates
- 1/2 cup raw cashews
- Zest of 1 lemon
- Juice of 1 lemon
- 2 tablespoons poppy seeds
- 1/4 cup shredded coconut, plus more for rolling

Instructions:

1. In a food processor, combine the pitted dates, raw cashews, lemon zest, lemon juice, poppy seeds, and shredded coconut.
2. Process until the mixture comes together and forms a sticky dough.
3. Roll the dough into bite-sized balls.
4. If desired, roll the energy balls in additional shredded coconut for extra coating.
5. Place the energy balls in an airtight container and refrigerate for at least 30 minutes to firm up.
6. Enjoy as a refreshing and energizing snack.

Chocolate Chip Oatmeal Cookies

Ingredients:

- 1 1/2 cups rolled oats
- 1/2 cup almond flour
- 1/4 cup maple syrup
- 1/4 cup melted coconut oil
- 1/4 cup almond butter
- 1/4 cup dairy-free chocolate chips
- 1 teaspoon vanilla extract
- 1/2 teaspoon baking powder

- 1/4 teaspoon salt

Instructions:

1. Preheat the oven to 350°F (175°C) and line a baking
    sheet with parchment paper.
2. In a bowl, combine the rolled oats, almond flour,
    maple syrup, melted coconut oil, almond butter,
    dairy-free chocolate chips, vanilla extract, baking
    powder, and salt.
3. Stir well until all the ingredients are evenly
    incorporated.
4. Drop spoonfuls of the cookie dough onto the
    prepared baking sheet and flatten them slightly with
    the back of a spoon.
5. Bake for 12-15 minutes, or until the edges are
    golden brown.
6. Remove from the oven and let the cookies cool on
    the baking sheet for a few minutes before
    transferring them to a wire rack to cool completely.
7. Enjoy these delicious, chewy cookies as a sweet
    treat.

Almond Butter Cups

Ingredients:

- 1/2 cup almond butter
- 1/4 cup melted coconut oil
- 2 tablespoons maple syrup
- 1/4 cup cocoa powder
- 1/2 teaspoon vanilla extract
- Pinch of salt

Instructions:

1. Line a mini muffin tin with paper or silicone liners.
2. In a bowl, combine the almond butter, melted coconut oil, maple syrup, cocoa powder, vanilla extract, and salt.
3. Stir until smooth and well combined.
4. Spoon a small amount of the almond butter mixture into each muffin cup, filling them about 1/3 full.
5. Place the muffin tin in the freezer for about 10 minutes to firm up.
6. Remove the muffin tin from the freezer and spoon the remaining almond butter mixture on top of each cup, filling them almost to the top.

7. Return the muffin tin to the freezer and freeze for at least 1 hour, or until the almond butter cups are solid.

8. Once frozen, remove the almond butter cups from the muffin tin and store them in an airtight container in the freezer.

9. Enjoy these homemade almond butter cups straight from the freezer whenever you crave a sweet and nutty treat.

Blueberry Crumble Bars

Ingredients:

Crust and Crumble Topping:

- 1 1/2 cups rolled oats
- 1 cup almond flour
- 1/2 cup coconut oil, softened
- 1/4 cup maple syrup
- 1 teaspoon vanilla extract
- Pinch of salt

Blueberry Filling:

- 2 cups fresh or frozen blueberries

- 2 tablespoons maple syrup

- 1 tablespoon lemon juice

- 1 tablespoon cornstarch

Instructions:

1. Preheat the oven to 350°F (175°C) and line a square baking dish with parchment paper.

2. In a bowl, combine the rolled oats, almond flour, softened coconut oil, maple syrup, vanilla extract, and salt for the crust and crumble topping.

3. Mix until the ingredients are well combined and form a crumbly texture.

4. Press two-thirds of the mixture into the bottom of the prepared baking dish to create the crust.

5. In another bowl, toss together the blueberries, maple syrup, lemon juice, and cornstarch for the blueberry filling.

6. Spread the blueberry mixture evenly over the crust in the baking dish.

7. Sprinkle the remaining oat mixture over the blueberry filling as the crumble topping.

8. Bake for 30-35 minutes, or until the top is golden brown and the blueberry filling is bubbling.

9. Remove from the oven and let cool completely in the baking dish.

10. Once cooled, cut into bars and serve as a delightful fruity dessert or snack.

Vegan Carrot Cake with Cream Cheese Frosting

Ingredients:

Cake:

- 2 cups grated carrots
- 1 1/2 cups all-purpose flour
- 1/2 cup almond flour
- 1 cup coconut sugar
- 1/2 cup melted coconut oil
- 1/4 cup unsweetened applesauce
- 1/4 cup almond milk
- 1 teaspoon baking powder
- 1/2 teaspoon baking soda
- 1/2 teaspoon ground cinnamon
- 1/4 teaspoon ground nutmeg

- 1/4 teaspoon salt

Cream Cheese Frosting:
- 1 cup vegan cream cheese
- 1/4 cup vegan butter, softened
- 2 cups powdered sugar
- 1 teaspoon vanilla extract

Instructions:
1. Preheat the oven to 350°F (175°C) and grease a round cake pan.
2. In a large bowl, combine the grated carrots, all-purpose flour, almond flour, coconut sugar, melted coconut oil, unsweetened applesauce, almond milk, baking powder, baking soda, ground cinnamon, ground nutmeg, and salt for the cake.
3. Stir well until all the ingredients are thoroughly mixed.
4. Pour the batter into the prepared cake pan and smooth the top with a spatula.
5. Bake for 30-35 minutes, or until a toothpick inserted into the center comes out clean.

6. Remove the cake from the oven and let it cool in the pan for 10 minutes.

7. Transfer the cake to a wire rack to cool completely.

8. Meanwhile, prepare the cream cheese frosting by beating the vegan cream cheese, softened vegan butter, powdered sugar, and vanilla extract together until smooth and creamy.

9. Once the cake has cooled, spread the cream cheese frosting evenly over the top.

10. Slice and serve this moist and flavorful vegan carrot cake to impress your friends and family.

Raspberry Coconut Bliss Balls

Ingredients:

- 1 cup dried raspberries
- 1 cup unsweetened shredded coconut
- 1/2 cup raw cashews
- 1/4 cup maple syrup
- 2 tablespoons coconut oil, melted
- 1 teaspoon vanilla extract
- Pinch of salt
- Additional shredded coconut, for rolling

Instructions:

1. In a food processor, combine the dried raspberries, shredded coconut, raw cashews, maple syrup, melted coconut oil, vanilla extract, and salt.

2. Process until the mixture forms a sticky dough and the ingredients are well combined.

3. Roll the dough into bite-sized balls.

4. If desired, roll the bliss balls in additional shredded coconut for coating.

5. Place the bliss balls in an airtight container and refrigerate for at least 30 minutes to firm up.

6. Enjoy these fruity and coconutty bliss balls as a healthy and satisfying snack.

Matcha Green Tea Popsicles

Ingredients:

- 2 teaspoons matcha green tea powder
- 1 can (13.5 ounces) coconut milk
- 1/4 cup maple syrup
- 1/2 teaspoon vanilla extract

Instructions:

1. In a bowl, whisk together the matcha green tea powder, coconut milk, maple syrup, and vanilla extract until smooth and well combined.

2. Pour the mixture into popsicle molds.

3. Place the popsicle molds in the freezer and freeze for at least 4 hours, or until the popsicles are completely solid.

4. Once frozen, remove the popsicles from the molds and enjoy these refreshing and antioxidant-rich treats on a hot day.

CONCLUSION

As we conclude this cookbook, we want to leave you with some final thoughts and encouragement. Remember that embracing a Vegan Diabetic Renal Diet is not a restrictive sentence but rather an opportunity to nourish your body and transform your relationship with food.

Be patient with yourself as you navigate this new way of eating. It's normal to face challenges and setbacks along the way. Embrace these as learning experiences and use them to refine your approach. Every day is a chance to make conscious choices that support your health and well-being.

Lastly, we would like to express our gratitude for choosing this cookbook as your companion on this journey. It has been an honor to guide you through the intricacies of a Vegan Diabetic Renal Diet. We hope that the knowledge and recipes shared have empowered you to take control of your health and discover the joy of delicious, plant-based meals.

As you step into the future, remember that you have the power to make a positive impact on your well-being through the choices you make. Embrace the nourishment, flavors, and variety that a Vegan Diabetic Renal Diet offers, and may it bring you vitality, balance, and renewed energy for years to come.

Wishing you health, happiness, and culinary adventures on your continued journey towards optimal health!